Living Well with Alzheimer's and Related Dementias

Moving & More

Care Facilities, Transitions, and Communication Basics

A Handbook for Caregivers

by

Jytte Fogh Lokvig, Ph.D.

Endless Circle Press
Santa Fe, New Mexico

"I may have Alzheimer's, but Alzheimer's doesn't have me."
- Brian LeBlanc

"I don't have Alzheimer's. I have part-timer's."
- Glen Campbell

"We desperately need others to see our abilities and not simply focus on our inabilities. Please enable us, don't further disable us."
- Myriam Marque, living with early onset Alzheimer's dementia

"I don't want to just survive. I want to live and thrive."
Laurie Scherrer, living with early onset Alzheimer's and FTD

"We desperately need the health care sector and the community to support us to live beyond the diagnosis of dementia…If you offer us proactive, rehabilitative and enabling post-diagnostic strategies for the disabilities that result from the symptoms of dementia, we can live better lives beyond diagnosis, and the pathway of loss, despair, and focus on our deficits will be reduced. We need to be enabled, not further disabled."
- Kate Swaffer and *John Sandblom*
Board members of the Dementia Alliance International living with dementia

Publication date: October 1, 2018
LIBRARY OF CONGRESS CONTROL NUMBER:
Pending

Drawings by the author

Endless Circle Press
228 Ojo de la Vaca Rd. Santa Fe, NM 87508
(505)466-8195
e-mail: EndlessCirclePress@gmail.com

Other books by Jytte Fogh Lokvig, Ph.D.

> Alzheimer's A to Z, Secrets to Successful Caregiving
> Alzheimer's A to Z, A Quick Reference Guide
> The Alzheimer's Creativity Project
> The Alzheimer's and Memory Café

Contents

Acknowledgments

I dedicate all my writings on living well with dementia and Alzheimer's to my dearest friend Bahtee Ames, whose grace and generosity of spirit inspired me to make this my life's work.

My work is inspired and encouraged by my many friends who are living with memory-impairment and who continue to demonstrate that dementia doesn't have to stand in the way of having a full and rich life. You continually remind me not to take anything for granted and you've taught me to let go of my own expectations and follow your flow and rhythm.

I also want to acknowledge the inspiration, encouragement, and support I receive from my many colleagues and friends in the national and international progressive eldercare movement, among them the Dementia Action Alliance, the Pioneer Network, The Santa Fe Healthcare Network, and the hundreds of you around the country who faithfully support Alzheimer's and Memory Cafes.

And to my friends and colleagues Karen Stobbe, Bill Thomas, Al Power, Susan Balkman, Kim McCrae, Karen Love, and many, many more - far too many of you to list on one page: Thank you so much; I'm privileged to know you and in awe of your compassion, strength, and generosity.

Meet Your Author

Dr. Jytte Fogh Lokvig is a nationally recognized Alzheimer's specialist with more than two decades of experience working with people living with neurocognitive degeneration, as well as families and caregivers. When an individual is living with dementia, family and friends are affected as well. Jytte's guidance helps everyone improve their lives by introducing them to the essentials in communication and effective approaches.

Lokvig works with care facilities, home care agencies and other organizations involved with people with dementia. She trains staff in dementia basics and uses her extensive experience in the arts and education to design programs that engage people in creative, stimulating, and enjoyable explorations, regardless of the severity of their dementia.

Dr. Lokvig works with local and international groups dedicated to progressive approaches to how we support our fellow beings living with cognitive impairment. One important component in this effort is the Alzheimer's (and Memory) Café movement. Dr Lokvig started the first Alzheimer's Café in North America in 2008 and maintains the national registry of cafés, numbering over 300 at the time of this writing.

My Dad was a youthful 80 year-old, when my brother and I attempted to have *the conversation* with him about his future if he found himself in need of assisted living or nursing care. The three of us visited a facility in his neighborhood. In the front lobby we passed a petite white-haired lady on her walker. Dad declared firmly (in Danish, his native tongue,) that he did not want to live in a place "where people come to croak!" He made us promise that he could stay forever in his home in San Diego. This turned out to be impossible.

For the next several years Dad summered with me in Santa Fe. An accomplished artist, he loved to spend his days in the city sketching the ancient pueblo architecture, so when it became apparent that he was no longer safe living by himself, I brought him up here to live with me. Things were fine for a couple of months when he announced to me that I was a really boring roommate and he needed to have more people around.

We found him a studio apartment at an assisted living facility in Santa Fe. It was the best decision we possibly could have made. Dad had his own friends and peers of his generation. I gave him my undivided attention when I was with him and when I was busy with my own life, I knew he was happy and safe.

The move had been my dad's decision; I was incredibly lucky. As I was to learn later, this is rarely the case, especially when the move is necessitated by the growing needs of the parent or loved one, especially those with some degree of memory loss. Even though Dad had initiated this, the move was still traumatic for him and I ended up spending a lot of time with him during the first month until he'd bonded with some of the other residents. Gentle transitioning is very important to our longterm success.

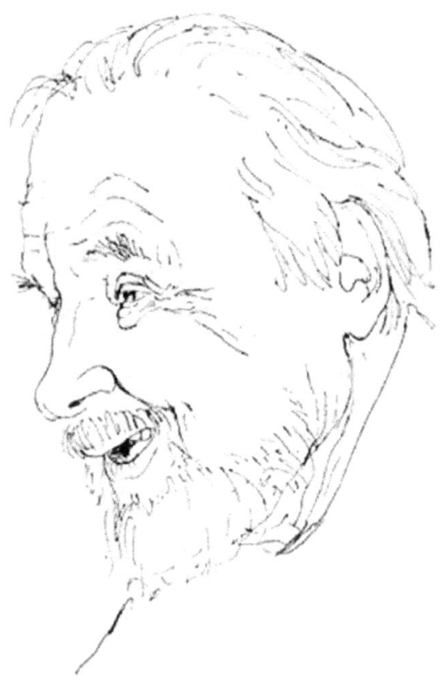

Aging-in-Place: The last decade has seen growing pressure for older people to "age-in-place" - to stay in their own homes till the end of life. This sounds ideal to many of us, but the realities of living alone for an elderly person are not quite as rosy as we'd like to believe. Most have had to give up driving, which means they are dependent on others for transportation. Maybe we made a solemn promise to our parents that they could live and die in their own homes. That was likely years ago before we were both faced with these realities: Mom can no longer clean her house; she's not eating right, she's forgetting to take her medications and because of her osteoporosis she's very vulnerable to injuries and falls. The biggest toll on her is likely to be her isolation. Loneliness is recognized as a major risk factor in this population, leading to depression, susceptibility to illness and early death. If she does remain at home, these are the realities we're facing:

Needs: Home care aides typically will provide personal care, such as showers, cooking, and light housekeeping; however, we cannot assume they will provide the social and intellectual stimulation necessary to a healthy mental state.

Cost: $20-30 per hour (through an agency)
24-hour care: $14,000 to $20,000 per month.

Relief and Respite

Caring for a person in your home brings its own hazards and the additional concerns of your own health and wellbeing. It's crucial that you take care of yourself. Even under the best circumstances, caregiving 24/7 is very stressful and puts caregivers at risk for physical and psychological repercussions.

Check with your community for services and programs that can bring relief, either for you or for both of you. For a start, many senior centers are safe places for someone in the earlier stages of dementia; aside from giving you, the caregiver, a much needed respite, the centers may offer inexpensive meals, fun classes, and other activities. These same centers may also run programs with volunteers, retirees or high school students, as companions or relief "sitters." Some locales have programs to provide you with free light housekeeping and handyman services. - - -

Every little bit helps, so take advantage of everything available.

Welcome to the Best Idea yet in Dementia Care. An Alzheimer's, Dementia or Memory café is a very "simple" concept: A monthly gathering of individuals with memory loss along with their caregivers, and/or friends and family in a safe, supportive, and engaging environment. The cafe gives everyone a welcome break from the disease.

Dr Bere Miesen started the first Alzheimer's Café in Leiden, The Netherlands in 1997. Dr. Lokvig opened the first café in the US in 2008 in Santa Fe, New Mexico.

When there's Alzheimer's or another dementia in the family, the disorder is a constant presence. Being out in public grows increasingly more stressful and yet it's important for people to feel part of their communities as long as possible. The café provides a respite in a judgment-free space with others who understand and share feelings. Many cafés bring in musicians and artists to share with the guests.

At the original café in Santa Fe, we always have creative projects on hand as well as our songbooks. The café is for people with dementia, including Alzheimer's, along with caregivers, families, friends, and professionals. Companions are expected to stay and participate in the café. The café will not exclude anyone based on age, race, color, religion, creed, or nationality. The café is a time to leave the disease at the door and just enjoy ourselves. The café is NOT: The café is not a support group, although it's likely to be the most supportive environment for everyone.

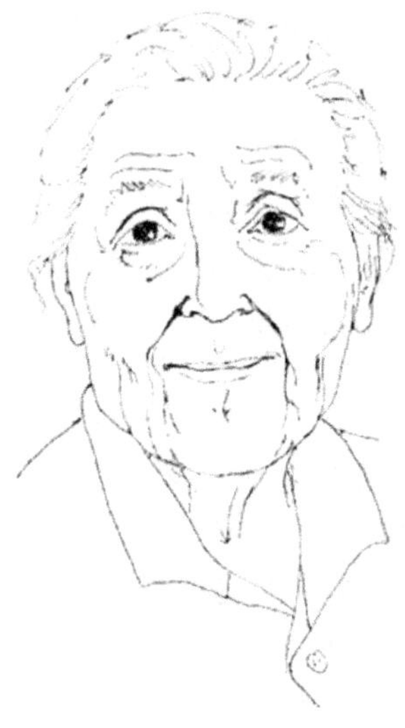

Support Groups

Support groups help you meet other caregivers. You'll have the opportunity to share ideas, suggestions . . . and tears. Check with organizations such as senior centers, AARP, the Parkinson's and Alzheimer's Associations, as well as local hospitals.

There are several different versions of shared care. Village to Village groups (http://www.vtvnetwork.org/) bring volunteers together to support and help individuals living at home ("aging in place") -   A similar approach is what we call "Share Care" - Caregiver support groups as well as Alzheimer's and memory cafés offer excellent opportunities to collaborate with others, and establish your own small "Share Care" group: Two, three or more of you join forces, visit at each others' homes, take in a movie, go on field-trips, share lunch at a cafe or go out for ice cream together. These shared experiences are not only pleasurable, but they help all of you to get to know each other, feel comfortable "sitting" for each other. This will make it easier to take respite breaks without worrying about your loved one.

The Promise

Does this sound familiar? Your loved one (your parent, spouse, friend) made you promise solemnly that you'd *never* let her go to a nursing home.

But now you realize that this was an unrealistic promise. It's clear that she's no longer the same person to whom you made that promise; she cannot care for herself. She's not eating right; the cartons from Meals on Wheels sit unopened in her refrigerator. She's subsisting on cereal and ice cream, losing weight and dehydrated which sometimes leaves her so unstable that you're seriously concerned about falls. - And since she and most of her friends no longer drive, they hardly ever get out to visit each other. So nowadays she spends her days alone, except when you have a chance to stop by.

It's time to face the fact that you simply cannot provide the support she needs now and the only realistic option is for her to move to a facility.

I strongly recommend that you start early and take your time to become familiar with longterm care options in your area. This process should not be rushed. I urge everyone who's caring for an elder at home to start this search long before it becomes a necessity and even if you think you'll never need it.

With the right approach on your part, this can be a totally positive move; the good news is that many people thrive when they move to a facility where they are with peers. I hope you'll take the time to familiarize yourself with all the options in your area. When you've narrowed your choices down to two or three, I recommend that you go back and spend at least a couple of hours and simply observe for a while. If you play "fly on the wall" it doesn't take long for people to forget you're there. Even if your loved one doesn't need it at this time, spend at least some of the time in "memory care." You're looking at interactions between residents, residents and staff, and staff with other staff.

This is what you want to see:

• Staff acknowledging all the residents, even with a simple brief greeting or compliment.

• Staff helping them get started on conversations, participating in their activities, however briefly, and never sounding condescending.

• NO babytalk EVER!!!! Everyone is an adult and deserves to be treated as such.

• Another red flag is staff discussing personal issues within earshot, especially if they are talking about residents.

Every state in the union has departments or offices that deal with issues relating to the elderly. Call your state's Agency on Aging, Health Department, Adult Protective Services or Ombudman's office. Ask questions, get information and learn of your state's licensing standards.

Independent living: Also known as retirement communities. Unregulated and unlicensed. Usually apartment-type complexes with the added conveniences of dining rooms and transportation. Some meals and light housekeeping are usually included in monthly fees.

Assisted living*: Usually state licensed. Included in monthly fees should be meals, personal hygiene, housekeeping, and laundry. Most assisted-living facilities have resident nurses to supervise and dispense medication.

Nursing homes*: Full nursing care available, federally regulated, and state licensed. Medicaid eligible. Often the only option for people with minimal resources.

Alzheimer's homes*: Full care for special-needs residents, state licensed. In some cases these homes are Medicaid eligible.

Continuing Care*: These residences offer all levels of care in a single facility, the theory being that this would allow a person to transition smoothly to a more advanced level of care. This works well as long as the facility makes a deliberate effort to integrate the populations and the activity programs.

* Facilities that are under the oversight of the Ombudsman program, a federally mandated resident advocacy agency.

The Eldercare Locator gives you a comprehensive overview of options in your area. They can also refer you to your local Agency on Aging (www.eldercare.gov or 800-677-1116, weekdays 9:00 am to 8:00 pm EST) as well as your local *Ombudsman**.

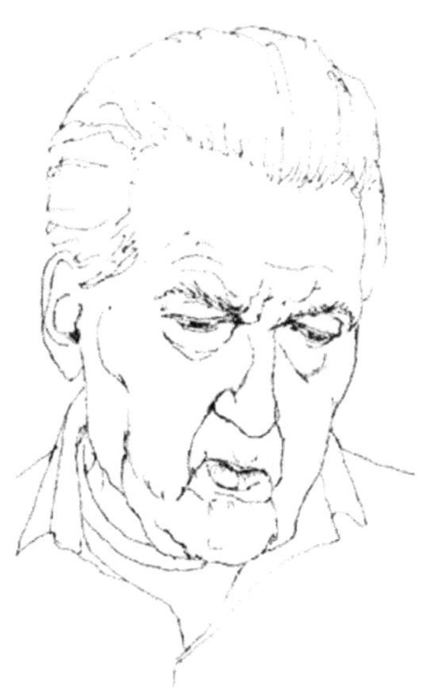

Start online, talk to other families, and call around. Once you have identified the facilities that you feel are possibilities for your particular situation, make appointments to tour the facility. I call this the "glamour tour" The marketing person's job is to impress you with all the exceptional features of the facility.

On this initial and all subsequent visits, look at it from the perspective of a resident. Typically, private pay facilities spend fortunes on the decor of the front lobby and the facade of the building to appeal to you, the customer. But nobody lives in the front lobby. You want to see the individual rooms or apartments that would be home for your loved one. Ask the marketing person to walk you to all the locations your loved one might frequent.

> What you want to learn on the tour:
> Does the facility practice "person-centered care"? Information on this concept can be found at the website for the Pioneer Network.
>
> **1.** Do residents choose what and when to eat and when they bathe?
>
> **2.** Do residents participate in menu and activity choices?
>
> **3.** Do residents have regular meetings.

4. What's the staff/resident ratio?

5. Staff retention rates?

6. Description of the staff-training program. (You want to hear that all staff receives mandatory first-aid and dementia training)

7. Who establishes residents' care-plans? (you want hear at least: family, nurse, personal care and activity staff.)

8. You want copies of menus and activities.

Be sure that you understand the financial aspects. Each facility is likely to have its own system, so be sure you get in writing all regular and additional potential charges.

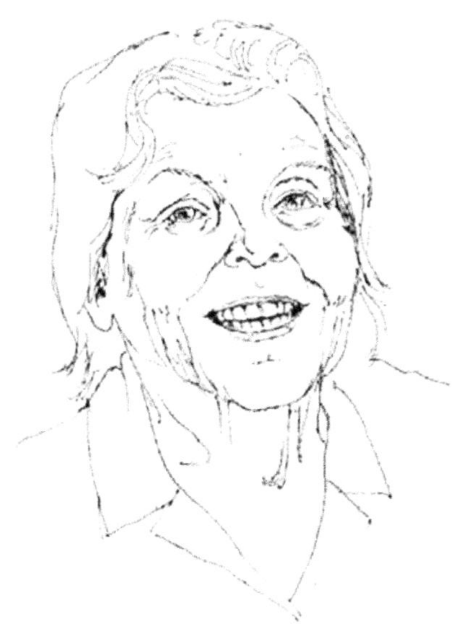

Once you've narrowed down your choices to three or four facilities, return on your own time to have lunch, talk to residents, and sit in on activities. Allow yourself a couple of hours at each facility; if this feels like a lot, please keep in mind that your loved one would be spending 24/7 in one of these communities. Of course you'll look at everything from your loved one's point of view, but your personal feelings are equally important. Could *you* envision living here? You'll be visiting a lot and you need to feel really good about the choice. If you are happy, the chances are better that your loved one will adjust sooner and be happy as well.

What to look for. On your follow-up visit observe interactions between residents and staff, resident to resident, and staff to staff. People with dementia and other brain disorders often have problems connecting to others. Ideally you'll see staff take a few seconds to initiate those contacts for them.

Food Services: Share at least one meal with residents in the dining room. Is the meal well-balanced and tasty? Are people offered alternatives to the day's entree? Are condiments readily available? Rather than impossible to open individual plastic packets, you'll want to see regular bottles or jars of mustard, catsup, and relish, as well as salt and pepper shakers and regional favorites. Are the residents offered seconds and plenty of liquid refills, both without having to ask? The residents should also have access to healthy snacks, fruits and nuts as well as drinks between meals. Observe the interaction between wait-staff and residents? Resident to resident?

Request a copy of the menu for the week. It should offer a well-balanced, and healthy diet with equally healthy alternative options. Does the menu reflect regional traditions as well of the choices of the residents?

If you're having a meal with residents in "memory care" chances are several of your table mates may have issues with perception, communication, and awareness. They might have forgotten how to use eating utensils or be confused by too many different types of food or simply too much on their plates. You'll want to see the staff step in to bring them relief. A staff can use the "hand-over" approach to guide a person's hand with a spoon or fork. If too much food on the plate confuses a person, he can be served the same food in small portions on a small plate.

Activities: Request a schedule of activities. A well-rounded program has a variety of offerings: Passive, active, and physical, intellectual, creative, and pure pleasure. There should also be a balance between group and individual activities. *Passive* activities are mostly pure entertainment, such as music performances, movies and games. Intellectually stimulating programs, i.e. lectures, classes, physical activities, and outings. And finally, the most important activities are not likely to be listed on the schedule. These are the individual projects that will be different for each resident. Regardless of people's cognitive abilities, it's crucial that they are supported in pursuing whatever gives them purpose and pleasure. This could be anything from setting the table, tending to the flower garden, painting or building clay sculptures.

Ask when and how the residents are encouraged to participate in the selection of activities, movies, and other aspects of the program. All too often, when we design programs, we rely on old standbys like Bingo. There's nothing wrong Bingo; it's a game and temporary entertainment for those people who are able to participate.

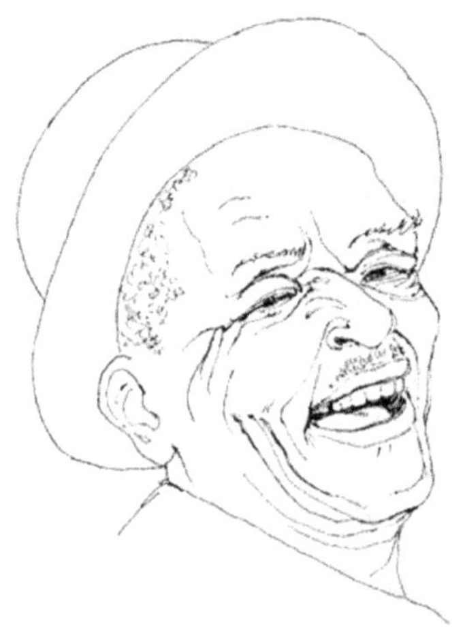

The Details

Now that you have chosen a facility for your loved one, it's time to make preparations. The more the staff knows about her habits and personality, the quicker she'll adjust to this being her home.

Quirks: Your loved one's interaction with staff will be a lot smoother if you share with them issues she has had lately, typically with personal care. - Be as specific as you can, even if it feels uncomfortable. Personal care is intimate and the more staff understands her particular quirks, the smoother their interaction with her will be.

Foods: List likes and dislikes she has around food. Her favorite foods and others she has rejected lately. It's tempting to insist to the staff that they serve her specific foods that you "know" she'll eat, but don't be surprised if her eating choices change in this new environment. She may feel freer to try new dishes in this new environment and she also may be influenced by other residents. Of course, you definitely want to list specifics about allergies, or other physical issues, i.e. missing teeth, which require easy to chew foods.

Sleep: Is she early to bed, early to rise? Or a night owl who loves sleeping in? Cool or warm room at night? How many hours does she usually sleep? Does she sleep through the night? - It's not unusual for people in later stages of dementia to have unstable body clocks, some even reversing day for night. In which case she needs purposeful activities at night.

Baths: Facilities typically offer two showers per week for each resident. If your loved one insists on more frequent showering you can expect to have added fees or to hire a private caregiver. Write out the routines that your loved one has been used to and comfortable with: Shower, tub, or neither? What time of day? Does she need privacy? Or is she okay with some assistance? Has she been washing her hair in the shower or does she usually go to a salon? - (Most private pay communities have salons.)

Personal care: How often does she see a podiatrist? A dentist? (Assuming she still has her own teeth.) Get a haircut? A manicure? The facility may provide some of these services, if not, you'll have to take care of them. There are more and more of these services being provided on a private pay "house-call" basic.

List any other personal hygiene or medical needs that you need the staff to be aware of.

Entertainment. What are her current preferences in movies, stories, songs and music, TV shows? Including what she definitely does not like.

History: A short biography will help staff relate and connect to your loved one. as well as a brief history of her life, focused on highlights that had made her happy, proud, and successful. If you're up to it, write all this up as anecdotes (short stories.) This way, staff can read them out loud. Everyone loves to hear about themselves.

Include pictures of parents, siblings, children, and best friends - with their names and a few facts, e.g. "Ruth, your aunt on your dad's side. She was the one with the tiny dog who thought he was a Great Dane" and "Cousin had bright red hair and loved chocolate mints"

I suggest that you create at least three copies - one for her chart, one for her room and one for you.

You've found a facility that you're pretty confident will work out for your mom. You may be fortunate enough that she has decided for herself that she's ready to move. But this is pretty rare and the majority of us are faced with a lot of resistance. You are determined to do all you can to make the move into her new environment as easy and as stress-free as possible, starting with not mentioning "moving" at all. The facility should be more than willing to support you in this transition program. In the long term, it saves them time and aggravation. The ideal is to introduce your loved one to the facility gradually. There shouldn't be any problems with management for the two of you to *visit* several times. (Explain the transition program to them.)

You can pretend to your loved one that you have both been invited to this *new* "café." When you talk to her about it, it's important that you treat your visits as regular outings. On your way there, talk with Mom as if it were just going to a new café: "Mom, we're gonna try a new place for lunch today. I hear they have good food and there are some really nice people there."

Make arrangements with management for you to sit with particular residents who have a special knack for making a newcomer feel welcome and at home.

And later, on the way home:

"I really enjoyed that lunch. The food was good, don't you think? And such nice people, especially that lady in the blue dress. She really liked you. You know, I'd like to go back again, wouldn't you?"

Feelings can't be rushed and it's worth as many visits as you need. In one case it took two months until one day my client said, "Can't I just stay here?" (Her apartment had been ready all along.)

Take your time. Usually it takes at least half a dozen such visits for a person to feel comfortable. These visits help her to make friends with other residents on her own terms, so when you move her in, everything is already familiar to her.

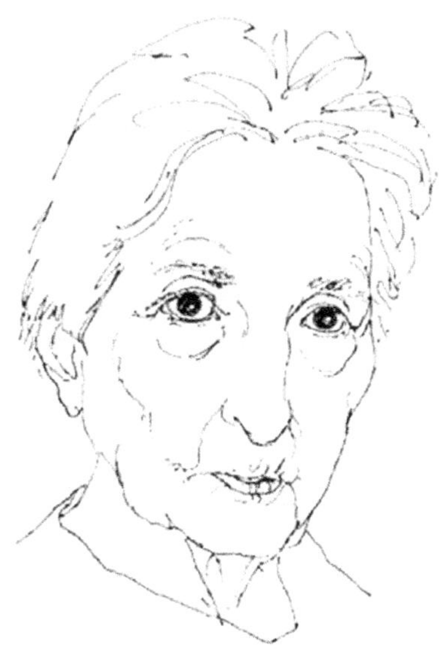

At these lunches, hopefully your loved one will soon feel at ease when other residents talk about their daily lives at the facility. Our temptation is to jump at the chance to push our loved ones, just a little, at this point. Please resist. As much as possible you want her to believe it's her choice. You have a better chance of success if you hold back and even when she brings it up, do not talk about her *living* there. *Living* is finite and permanent and could be frightening to her. Instead talk about her possibly "staying" for a while. *Staying* is not specific. It could mean an hour, a week or ten years. Words matter.

At some point, you might say something along these lines: "Mom, I hate to tell you this, but we'll have to get going now, but it sure would be so nice to spend more time here, don't you think?" Consider variations of this approach and then increasingly build on the idea of staying there. Then when it feels right, you can try this:

"I'm sorry we had to leave so soon. I know you'd like to spend more time with your friends, wouldn't you? You know, they really like you and they seem sad every time you have to leave. I wonder if they might have a room there for you. Wouldn't that be great? Then you'd be close to your friends all the time. This is a very popular place, so they don't often have vacancies. But we can ask, right? Cross your fingers."

And then finally, the day before her move, be really excited: "I have the best news for you! I just got a phone call and they're saving one of their best rooms for you. Isn't that exciting? I told them that you'd be very happy to hear that. We'd better jump on it before they give it to someone else. Come on, let's celebrate!"

On moving day, take her to the facility in the morning and let her mingle with her friends while you discreetly move her belongings in. Be sure her pictures and possessions are in place before you bring her to into her room. Walk her in as if it were the executive suite at a four star hotel:

"Welcome to your room, Mom. Boy, aren't we lucky that this was available? Isn't it nice? Look at this great view (if it has one) and see how lovely your pictures look in here."

Sit down with her in her new place and have a normal and casual conversation. She'll see how comfortable you feel being there and that will help her get over any possible anxiety. Stay with her until her bedtime and try to have breakfast with her the following morning. If she gets very anxious at this point, you may have to spend the night with her.

For the next few weeks, join her for as many meals and activities as you can. You can gradually taper off to a reasonable number of visits. It's very important to let her know that you want to spend time with her there and that you'll continue to do so.

If your loved one is living in the "secure" (locked) dementia wing, it's particularly important that you happily share in her experiences and life there. Some facilities give family members the option to take their loved one up to the "assisted living" dining room; it's usually a nicer set-up. To me, this sends the wrong message that you don't like the dementia wing. So, I ask you how can we expect our loved ones to flourish in their environment if we escape it whenever we have the chance?

It sounds like a lot of work, and it is, but taking the time now will save you the stress you'd no doubt go through if Mom were moved in without any preparation at all.

Keep in mind that a care facility is a shared environment. Things can be misplaced, forgotten, broken or mixed up with someone else's stuff. There are certain preparations that can spare you future aggravations. Don't let this list scare you. This may be being overly cautious because no large community, even the grandest hotel, is one hundred percent secure.

- Leave anything at home, that can't be replaced, such as beloved breakable knick-knacks, or precious paintings.
- If your mom loves her jewelry, you'll have to decide whether it's worth the risk to bring them. An alternative is to find similar costume jewelry and to leave the real stuff in the safe.

- Mark her clothes and linens with her name in washable ink or you can purchase iron-on laundry proof custom labels - several options available online.

- If she wears glasses, mark them as well. This is tough, because obviously there's no place to attach a label. I found a workable solution: Painting several coats of nail polish on the inside of the temple stems –

- If you wish to do so, it's legal for you to install granny-cams in her room.

Tip for the facility:
- If several residents use prescription glasses, you can personalize these markings by using a different color nail polish or model paint for each resident, i.e. all blue belongs to Marie, while all green belongs to Sally.

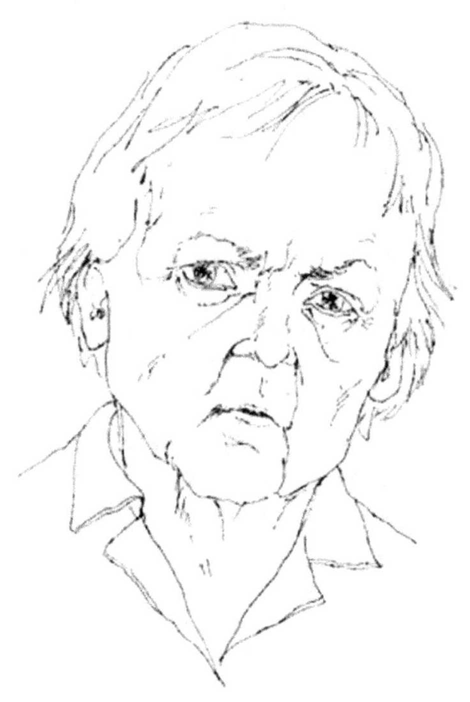

The first week. Now that she's *staying* here, there are things you can do to support her and help make this transition smoother and easier. During the first several days, try to spend as much time as possible with her, participating in meals and activities, including at least one shower, possibly staying over for a few nights.

In some cases, it works better for you not to be involved in the actual move. The reason: Some of us still fare racked with guilt and can't get over feeling guilty at moving our loved one into a facility. It's important that this move is a very positive experience and since it's very hard to hide our feelings, it may be better to have a family friend or caregiver at your loved-one's side and let her settle in before bringing you back into the picture.

Your team: You and the staff share a common goal: to do the very best for your loved one. It may be hard at times, if she's telling you that she has all kinds of problems. Some complaints may be legitimate, while others may be exaggerations, hallucinations or delusions, based on her confusion, so before we jump to conclusions and accuse someone of wrong-doing, let's take a deep breath. The staff is usually the best source for a truthful accounting.

This is the most common complaints that you'll hear from a person who's new to the community:

Someone is stealing from her. She claims someone stole her purse. This happens a lot when a resident has forgotten where she left it.

Or she screams at you that someone is going through her apartment and stealing her things. It's tempting to tell her that she's mistaken and all her precious belongings are in safekeeping at your house. However, she'd most likely accuse you of lying. Before you panic and allow yourself to succumb to guilt and second-guessing your decision to move her in here, take a deep breath and tell her calmly that you'll check into the situation right away. And then find a good distraction, a cup of tea, a walk outside, or a good magazine.

There will be times when you suspect something may actually have gone wrong. Talk to the staff about what your loved one alleges happened. Remember they are your allies.

Attitude: Your own feelings and attitude are crucial to your success. As much as you can, participate along with your loved one with enthusiasm, without going overboard. Eat with her, create with her, and join her in conversations with other residents. When she observes you so accepting of her new life, it will help her feel at home sooner.

Patience: Get to know individual staff members and work with them. You are all on the same team. They have many other residents to care for in addition to your loved one, and are often overwhelmed. In my experience, longterm staff are people who have chosen to stay in this field because they want to make a difference in someone's life, - definitely not for the money. It's demanding work, underpaid and under-appreciated. So, please be patient with them and let them know you appreciate what they do.

Many of us are so relieved that our intense search is over and we've found a place for our loved ones and we can sleep through the night, knowing they are safe.

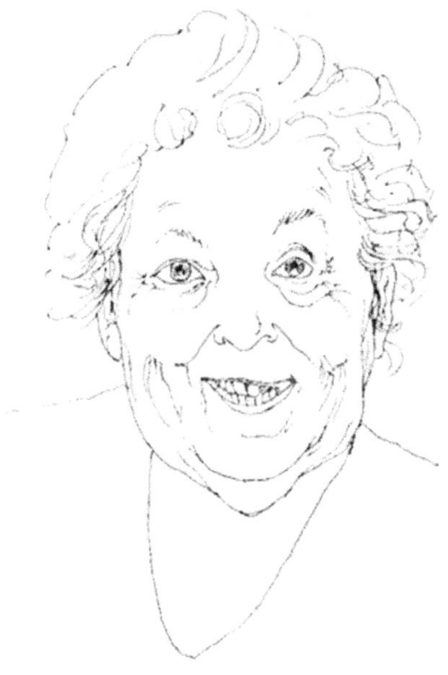

Welcome to the World of
Alzheimer's and Dementia

In 1994, when I first got involved with the Alzheimer's and dementia community, there was very little conversation and information outside the specific medical establishment. This has changed. Dementia has become a regular feature in popular media. Alzheimer's in particularly is now used as the big bad monster that destroys everything in its path. I find this most disturbing. Alzheimer's is only one of hundreds of brain disorders sharing the symptoms of dementia, no worse and no better, albeit the most prevalent by far.

Unlike physical disabilities, dementia, including Alzheimer's, has no outward signs to the casual observer. A person can appear "normal" most of the time even when he's struggling with his daily life getting increasingly more confusing and overwhelming. It's particularly difficult for those closest to him to accept and understand what is happening to his brain. He may have moments when he forgets names of his own family members. This is devastating for everyone. It's tempting to think that he's being ornery or stubborn when in fact it's the disease causing a mental block.

We all think about our retirement years and what our life will be like as we get older. I know I did, I thought I would end up on some beach in the south. I planned ahead and thought I had all my ducks in a row until I got the results telling me I had dementia, probably of the Alzheimer's type.

All my ducks scrambled, and my life got turned around. I spent the next 14 years trying to get those duck back in a row and get control over my life once again. I found I was turning into a different person living in a different world.

I was angry that my life was being taking away and feared what the future held for me. I gave up my life to a higher power and started to learn how to live in this new world of dementia.

Here I am after those 14 years of learning, happier then I thought I ever could be. I may not be on the beach in the South, but I sit on my bench under a beautiful sky enjoying this wonderful life I created.

I was given a passion of teaching others to follow my lead of a life after your diagnosis. You can be happy regardless what the book tells you. This new world we are entering is beautiful if you get rid of the old baggage you are carrying and see life the way it really is.

Harry Urban

A very, very short primer

"Dementia" is not a specific disease. It's a term used to describe **symptoms** shared by hundreds of brain disorders: Memory and thinking problems severe enough to affect a person's ability to perform everyday activities.

- **Alzheimer's Disease** - Identified by amyloid plaques and neurofibrillary tangles. Most common dementia; accounts for an estimated 60 - 80 percent of all dementia cases.

- **Vascular Dementia** – Also known as multi-infarct, post-stroke dementia, or vascular cognitive impairment

- **Mixed Dementia** - Characterized by the hallmark abnormalities of Alzheimer's along with another type of dementia

- **Dementia with Lewy Bodies** - (LBD) Similar to Alzheimer's. Hallucinations are common.

- **Parkinson's Disease** - People with Parkinson's disease often develop dementia in the later stages of the disease.

- **Frontotemporal Dementia (FTD)**– Affects personality, judgment, and reasoning.

- **Pick's disease** – One type of frontotemporal dementia.

- **Creutzfeldt-Jakob Disease** – In some cases known as Mad Cow disease (variant Creutzfeldt-Jakob Disease)

Delirium. The following conditions may mimic dementia, but are often reversible:

- **Normal Pressure Hydrocephalus** (NPH) - Buildup of fluid in the brain; may be *reversible.*

- **Dehydration**

- **Malnutrition**

- **Infections** (very common: UTIs or urinary tract infection)

- **Drug reactions**

- **Drug interactions**

- **Reactions to anesthesia**

The physical and chemical changes in the brains of people with dementia, including Alzheimer's, affect comprehension and memory as well as mood, energy and spirit. The individual is more susceptible to outside stimuli and has less control over his emotions. When we experience sadness or grief, most of us are able to reason ourselves out of our blues and our strong feelings fade pretty quickly.

People living with dementia typically lose their abilities to interpret their feelings. Thus, their negative feelings last a lot longer, often unchanged in intensity. Sadness and anger tend to linger longer than happy and joyful feelings. With that in mind, we can see the importance of maintaining a positive attitude and understanding how to guide people into a better space.

It's one thing to understand logically what's happening when our loved ones are depressed or angry, quite another to deal with our own emotions. Outbursts can feel like personal attacks, and yet it's important not to take any of them personally. As the saying goes: "It's the dementia acting out." Often outbursts are caused by a loss of self-determination, purpose, and a sense of powerlessness.

This important piece of advice sounds a lot easier than it is for most of us:

DON'T REACT TO ATTACKS,
don't justify or explain, or try to reason
and above all,
DON'T DISAGREE OR ARGUE!

Reacting or arguing will only escalate and prolong the conflict. Instead, change the conversation to something positive and unrelated to the subject of the rage. When his outburst happens out of the blue, you may want to validate his anxiety with a simple remark: "It sounds like you're really upset." But before his agitation escalates even more, offer him a distraction. This could be a bowl of ice cream, a walk, - or an activity. He may need an ego-booster right now, so whatever you choose, find something on which you can compliment him. Anything that needs to be sorted out works particularly well in these situations. Hand him a *fiddle box** and say, "See what I just found. You're much better than me at sorting stuff; would you mind looking at this?"

If this is a particularly intense confrontation - or if your attempt to distract him fails, pretend that you must use the bathroom immediately and exit the room. A few minutes later return with a big smile and positive demeanor as if you just arrived and are really happy to see him.

A typical scenario: He mentions a particular gadget and yells at you, *"Where is it? It's mine! You stole it!"* He threw out this particular item out years ago, but if you try to convince him of that, he won't believe you and you'll probably only agitate him even more. Instead, you may answer like this, *"I'm right in the middle of something, but if you can wait a few minutes I'll be glad to help you look for it. - While I finish up here, would you mind holding this box for me?"* You have giving him validation, but immediately distracted him with something to do: holding a *fiddle box*.* Most likely his curiosity will take over and he'll start *fiddling* with the contents.

*The *fiddle box* has consistently been our most effective tool: a shoe box or similar container filled with a perfusion of odds and ends of items that can be sorted, counted, lined up or simply looked at untouched. It's important that the fiddle box looks messy.

Another scenario: You left the room for a few minutes and when you return, he greets you with a tirade: *"Where have you been? Why did you leave me here all alone? You said you'd be right back. You lied."*

People with Alzheimer's and other dementias often lose the sense of time and space; when you've been out of sight, he may not be able to gauge how long you've been gone. Two minutes may feel like an hour to him. However trying to "set him straight" is an exercise in futility. Instead, you may simply say, *"I'm sorry I took so long. I'm so glad you waited for me. Thank you. (And then the diversion:) – I could use a snack right about now. You want to keep me company?"*
In both of these scenarios you've deflected his anxiety without reminding him of his memory loss or accusing him of lying. Thus you have maintained his dignity. As much as possible use compliments and let him know that you're happy to be there with him. With practice, this approach will become second nature to you.

Words Matter
With and about people living with
dementia, including Alzheimer's

The following lists were compiled by people living
with dementia, including Alzheimer's.

• Don't blame me for the changes in my behavior or
personality.

• Don't assume I can't answer for myself.

• Don't talk about me to someone else, in front of me.

• Don't assume we can't communicate even if we can't
speak.

• Don't assume we don't understand just because
we are silent.

• Don't assume because we can't tell you, your
words or actions don't hurt our feelings.

On the other hand, dementia, including Alzheimer's,
can teach the rest of us to simply to BE and appreciate
each other as unique individuals with something to
contribute, big or small. Whether we're family
members, personal aides, doctors, nursing or
activity staff, we can let go of our roles and lend
ourselves to the persons we're with.

INAPPROPRIATE TERMS

We don't identify people by their disorders or diseases: i.e. If we have chronic conditions like diabetes or scoliosis, we wouldn't want to be referred to as a diabetes person or scoliosis person, would we? How would we feel if these words were used about us?

Alzheimer's person, Demented person should be "A person living with Alzheimer's or dementia"

Crippling, Demented, Victim, Sufferer, Invisible, Fading, Not all there, Empty shell, Losing it - - - These terms assume that we should use our own standards to judge others. Well, in that case, whose standards? - yours or mine?

Behavior problem, challenging behaviors, difficult behaviors. Often the "problem" is with the caregiver and a lack of understanding communication. A person who has lost his ability to communicate with words will resort to other ways. If he's frustrated that you don't get the urgency of his problem, he may flail, gesture, make loud noises or even strike out. We call this "behavioral expression." - What would we do if we were stuck in a foreign country and needed help but didn't know the language?

Vocalizer, Aggressor, Wanderer, Sundowner, Feeder. We don't describe each other by our actions, so why do so with people with dementia? We have stripped them of their humanness.

Fighting Alzheimer's, War on Alzheimer's, Win over or beat Alzheimer's, Battling Alzheimer's. Combative terms keep us in a negative and often hopeless state. Until we come up with a cure, Alzheimer's and other dementias are chronic conditions and for everyone's sake, let's make the best of our situations.

And lastly *The long goodbye.* Pleeeeeeease!!! This may be the most cruel of all. Does this mean that a person starts dying as soon as he is diagnosed? In that case, we could legitimately start using that term with any newborn infant, because the truth is we're all dying a little every day of our lives.

So, to borrow from Richard Taylor who lived well for over ten years with a diagnosis of dementia, probably of the Alzheimer's type: "I'm still **ME**, so let's say **HELLO**"

The Basics

Good advice in any relationship,
but especially in the case of dementia.

Listen!

Avoid: "Do you remember?"

USE WITH CARE: "DO YOU WANT?"

Avoid the word **"NO!"**

Avoid Baby Talk -it's condescending

Use compliments and humor
(a lot, - but never at your companion's expense)

NEVER ARGUE, SCOLD OR CRITICIZE

Use **Diversions** and Loving Lies

Respect **altered** realities

ASK FOR HELP

Join in a laugh as often as possible

Communication

Two minutes now will save thirty minutes later.

I was early for a training session with the staff at a large nursing home, so I decided to wait in the lunchroom. Several residents were still eating, while half a dozen who had finished were lined up in their wheelchairs waiting to be escorted back to their rooms. One woman in a wheelchair was off by herself, crying loudly, "Help, help, help me." An aide rushed past her, close enough to brush up against her arm. Several other staff were eating their lunches at a corner table.

I watched this scenario for a while. The staff was oblivious to her cries and it was soon apparent that nobody would do anything, I went to the unhappy resident's side, asked her name and how I could help. She told me she was afraid to be left behind, so I wheeled her to the back of the line of the wheelchair line and reassured her that someone would help her in a few minutes. She smiled, relaxed into her chair and closed her eyes for a quick nap.

This woman's outcries were likely such a frequent and annoying occurrence that the staff had conditioned themselves to ignore her. However, when one person is obviously upset like this, it affects everyone else around her. There's often a snowball effect in these situations. One person's loud outcries can cause agitation in others, which in turn can affect their interactions with staff. It would have been so easy for the staff person to give her a few seconds of her attention, thus putting her at ease, which would help everyone have a much better afternoon, the residents and staff alike.

Listen

A person with more advanced dementia may have aphasia (impairment of language) making it difficult for him to form words and sentences; however this does not necessarily indicate diminished comprehension or reasoning. So when he mutters something, take a deep breath and concentrate on what he's trying to say and simultaneously to what his body language is telling you. He may know exactly what he means and understandably get upset when his babbling is ignored. Hard as it may be for us, he still deserves our undivided attention for a few minutes. Help him with a non-specific response to validate his opinion.

It's even more challenging to interact with him when he has lost his speech altogether. At that point we need to be much more proactive and observant, paying close attention to his body language and to continue to include him in decisions and conversations. It makes a big difference to his quality of life when we talk through any actions that affect him.

Caregiving involves performing tedious routines on a daily basis. Under those circumstances it's hard to remember that while these may be routine to us, to a demented person each time may be a new and scary experience. For example if she is in a wheelchair, you likely move it several times during the day and it may be hard to remember that each move may be startling to her. After all, she ought to be used to it. However, can you imagine how it feels to have "the rug" yanked out from under you? Try it sometime. Sit in a wheelchair and have someone move you without warning – it feels very insecure and I suspect a person never really gets used to it. So, please make a habit out of talking through your actions to let the person know what you're going to do. It can be a brief remark: "I need to move your chair, okay?"

Tell her a moment before when you need to take other actions that may alarm her, i.e. straightening out blankets, pillows or bedding; putting on or removing a piece of clothing or shoes; buttoning something; giving her another spoonful of food, combing her hair or wiping her hands.

Eye contact. Always approach from the front. If your resident is snoozing or appears to be off in her own world, you may need to get her attention. Lean down to eye level and gently tap her knee. Before you say or do anything else, make eye contact with her to gain her full attention. This is especially important when you need her cooperation with a specific action, such as changing her clothes, giving her medication or brushing her teeth.

Catherine never wanted to burden anyone with her problems, so she would try her best to avoid anything relating to herself. Unfortunately she was prone to frequent urinary tract infections (UTI) that can lead to other serious infections, so it was important for us to know when we needed to intervene before the infection spread. We got used to paying close attention to Catherine's body language. Her appetite, demeanor and movements would change even if the topics of her conversations did not.

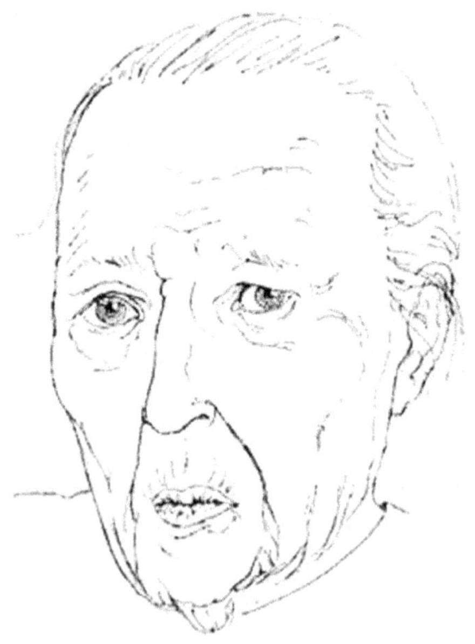

Baby Talk

It's normal for human beings to change our voices into a higher register and softer tones to express sympathy and compassion. However, it may be hard for us to distinguish between compassion and condescension. What may be meant as an expression of concern or simple kindness, can sound quite demeaning. Unfortunately I've often witnessed this kind of unconscious condescension from both staff and visitors.

> *Just imagine yourself on the receiving end*
> *of cutesy tones and baby talk.*

Example: Three of us were sitting side-by-side, relaxing in easy chairs after lunch: One of the residents in the dementia care wing, flanked by me on one side and her husband on the other. The facility's marketing person was giving a tour to a few people. One of the visitors bent down in front of the husband and very sweetly said, "*Hi, how are you?*" The visitor's tone of voice clearly suggested that she thought the husband was an impaired resident as well. A little too sweet and condescending. She meant well, trying to *connect* with a person she assumed to be disabled because of the circumstances and his appearance. He was perfectly lucid, but had a mane of white hair and a handsome man with wrinkles appropriate for someone in his late eighties. Most of us have a tendency to change our tone with someone we perceive as being weak and vulnerable. So, the point is not so much that the visitor was mistaken but rather that she didn't realize that nobody wants to be considered an object of pity, as the visitor's tone had suggested, even in advanced stages of dementia.

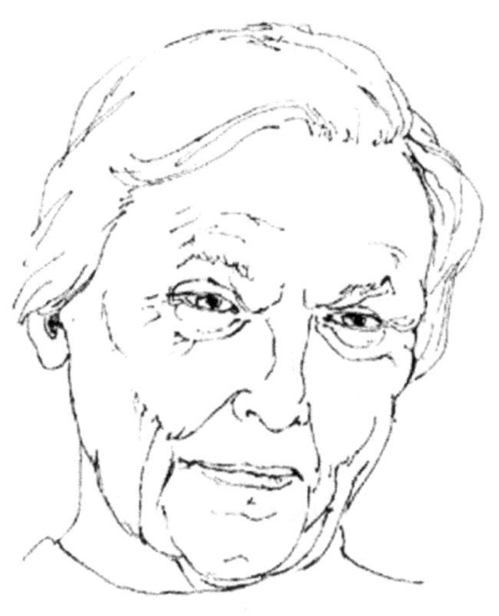

Compliments

I'm sure you would agree that the world would be a gentler and kinder place if we would spend less energy on criticizing and more on complimenting each other on our strengths. It's so easy to greet everyone with a short remark to boost their spirits. "Geraldine, that shirt is such a good color for you." "David, so glad you could make it today. It's not the same without you." It's about recognizing our unique personhood and acknowledging how important we are to each other. Compliments should be in every visitor and caregiver's bag of tricks. You can stop an unwanted behavior or reaction with a compliment and you can help a person out of her funk by talking about her unique talents. You may even be able to get her into the shower by complimenting her on how well she has always taken care of herself (even if it's been years since this was the case;) You may want to add that you'll do your best to live up to her standards.

Rosamund was a perfectionist and when things didn't go well for her, she would get very upset with herself. Her agitation soon affected the whole group. We got used to diverting her by asking her to help sort something out. In her case it always worked, because we could be totally sincere when we'd say, "Rosamund, you are the best organizer and I really could use your help."

Humor

Dementia causes people to lose their memory and they may be confused about a lot of things in their lives, however they generally retain a healthy sense of humor - provided they had one in the first place. Laughter's really good for our health, and it's crucial for anybody involved in caregiving, whether giving or receiving. Laughter, giggles, and chuckles are healthy for us because they help us relax, improve our heart health and take the pressure off when folks have difficulty expressing themselves. Try to infuse your daily routines with a light spirit. You'll find that the most fluid conversations happen when people are paying attention to something other than themselves and a funny story will do that. It's particularly important that we laugh at ourselves. I maintain a growing collection of funny sayings and jokes. This material comes in handy when I've needed an instant diversion. Favorites over many years have been *Stupid Laws* and quotes from folks like *Zsa Zsa Gabor* and *George Burns*.

I suggest that you go online and search for some of these: Google search: "Funny." You'll find funny quotations, hilarious real classified ads, and many more goodies. One of my own favorites is "Disorder in the Courts," a collection of actual exchanges in court proceedings, from record compiled by court reporters. (Go to Resources)

Arguing does not work. Period! This is true in all relationships, but it's particularly true in our relationships with people made vulnerable by dementia. There's no way a memory-impaired person can hold up his end in an argument, so his choices are limited to withdrawing into a shell, becoming agitated or even striking out physically. It's counterproductive of course and it most likely will escalate your issues because it's doubly difficult to pull a person out of his withdrawn or agitated state.

Admonishing, criticizing, or correcting someone is demeaning and insulting. Just like arguing pushes a person away from you, admonishing will widen the gulf between you and make your task doubly difficult.

"Don't do that." an auto-response that's very hard for us to drop. Even if your resident is pouring her milk all over her fish filet, plate and table, try to find a response other than this admonishment. - And be aware that she may have no idea what you're referring to when you say: **"Don't do that."** Instead, you can offer to pour the milk off her plate and into a bowl or a cup. Hard as it is, keep your tone calm, as though this was a perfectly normal thing to do.

Sharing memories without pushing buttons

Asking a memory-impaired person this question is like asking a vision-impaired person, "You see this?" If you start a conversation with: "Do you remember?" – the response may be "No" or simply a blank stare. It stands to reason that this question might put off a person with memory issues and bring the conversation to an abrupt halt. All you were trying was to have a pleasant reminiscence. You had a particular shared experience in mind. There's absolutely nothing wrong with wanting to share a memory, but instead of asking a direct question, start talking about your own memories of that experience. If your story appears to bring pleasure, you can retell it repeatedly, perfecting your storytelling technique in the process. The beauty of advanced dementia is that it allows your listener to have wonderful experiences over and over again through your narrations, especially when she's a central character in the tale.

In my opinion we put too much stock in memories and academic knowledge - and not enough in imagination. You may have heard the saying: *without your memory, you're nothing*. This is so not true. A person with Alzheimer's still retains his personhood although he may appear changed to those around him. There's typically a tipping point in the disease when he has lost so much of his memory that he's able to live in the moment and may have the time of his life. It gives us the opportunity to make up wonderful new stories and draw on his imagination.

Connie was aware that her memory was terrible, so she took me aback when she suggested that we hold a lecture series. When I asked about suggestions for specific subjects, she said she didn't care; it could be anything, she just wanted to hear something serious, real, and grown-up. I think we need to remember that some of us may recall specifics for years while others like Connie will forget almost immediately but that does not mean that we don't all deserve intellectual and mental stimulation.

Use with care: "Do you want?"

Choices are good. Choices help boost a person's self esteem, but a memory-impaired person may need to **see or touch** the choices. A good way to start the day is holding up two shirts and ask, "Which one would you like to wear? This red one or the blue one?" She can then simply point to her choice and you can throw in a bonus compliment, "Excellent choice. This color is so good on you; it makes your eyes sparkle."

Many facilities offer menus with a couple of alternatives of entrees. That's a good thing. The problem arises when wait-staff takes orders as much as an hour before the meal is served. By the time the plates arrive, the residents have completely forgotten what they had ordered in the first place. Staff can easily eliminate this problem by showing the actual plates and letting the residents pick which one they want.

It's virtually impossible to eliminate the use of "do you remember?" and "Do you want?" Both are ingrained in our language, so rather than beat yourself up when you've slipped, develop a habit of looking for reactions. When you see that vacant and lost gaze of not understanding, repeat your question as an anecdote with an explanation.

Avoid using "NO!"

When a vulnerable person makes a high-risk move, many of us would automatically yell at her to stop with a loud "**NO!**" It's risky when it involves a confused individual. Her action likely makes perfect sense to her, so if you yell "**STOP!**" or "**NO!**" she may have no idea *what* she's supposed to stop. Unfortunately this reflex reaction on our part will often aggravate the situation.

Elvira was still in the earlier stage of dementia. Very early in my career, before I knew any better, I came to see her in her small apartment. She usually handled herself really well, so I didn't think anything of it when she stepped into her kitchenette to make us a cup of tea. We were chatting; I watched from the breakfast bar as she filled the kettle and turned on the stove. That's when things started going haywire. Instead of the kettle, she put a potholder on the burner. My insides screamed *"NO, NO, NO!"* but fortunately instincts kicked in; instead I flew into the kitchen, yanked the flaming potholder off the burner and pitched it into the sink, while I put my arm around her shoulders and with all the calm that I could muster, I changed to subject away from tea, kettles and gas burners.

"No" runs the risk of achieving one or two things right away: alienating or pushing a person away or even worse, it can startle her so that she can't think straight and may exacerbate the action you were trying to halt.

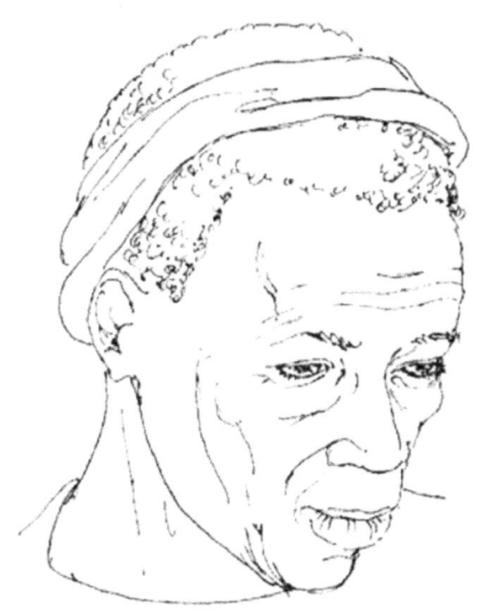

There are times when you need an instant diversion, because the situation is not likely to be resolved by your trying to reason with her, i.e. She's suddenly agitated for no reason that's apparent to you.

> *First* do not contradict or argue with her.
> *Acknowledge and delay:* "I'd be glad to help you right after we've had lunch (or made the bed, finished the dishes, taken the trash out.)"
> *Ask for help* (folding clothes, sorting mail)

Exception: If your most irresistible activity fails to distract her for anymore than a few minutes, her agitation may have a physical origin. She could be hungry, tired, or have a low-grade infection.

Maggie insists that someone has stolen her money. You've already tried to tell her that her daughter handles all her money – But your explanation only makes Maggie more agitated and insistent that it's her money and she wants you to take her to the bank to get it *right now*! Instead of trying to convince her that it's safe in the bank, try this: Tell her: "I'll be glad to help you right after I've finished here." (make up a task if you need to) and then add: "I sure could use your help with this." Then find her a diversion that will occupy her and change the conversation to take her mind off her money.

Altered reality is the term I use when a resident is reliving the past, usually the distant past. These events are typically thought of as *hallucinations*. As a person loses her short-term memory and most of her other more recent recollections are too fractured to make sense to her, the only memories that are somewhat intact are usually from her childhood and very early adulthood. When she slips into one of these early memories, her experience is different from ours.

She's not remembering the way most of us recall something. We are aware that this is a memory of an event that occurred some time ago, but to her it's happening right now. Alzheimer's or dementia has changed her perception of time and space. She relives her memory with as much veracity as she experiences the here-and-now. The present and the past overlap and commingle. Very often these time slips happen without warning. From observations over the years, I feel that these shifts into altered realities happen particularly at these times:

- Something in her environment disturbs her.
- Her body clock has been activated.
- She's hungry, tired, scared, bored, or aching.

It's counterproductive to try to convince her that she's *just remembering* something. Instead, join in her experience to connect with her or help her if she's reliving something disturbing. Remember that this is *her* reality and your *loving lie* is her truth at the moment.

Marge had just been moved to the "Alzheimer's wing" from upstairs in the facility. No attempts had been made to help her to transition from the freedom of her own apartment into this restrictive environment. She recognized right away that it was a locked/secure unit and she was understandably upset. By mid-afternoon she was at the locked door trying in vain to work the code on the keypad. When her attempts failed she started pounding on the door and yelling for someone to open it. She finally collapsed into a pile on the floor, sobbing.

It's pretty common for newcomers to be very upset in these new and unfamiliar surroundings, if they have not had proper transitioning. So staff didn't think much of it. They tried to calm her down and coerce her back into the common room with no luck. Finally two aides dragged her away from the door. Once they had her seated, it took considerable time and effort from both of them to calm her down.

During the day Marge continued to adjust quite well. However, by mid-afternoon she was back at the locked door and her agitation didn't diminish. Because the outbursts happened in the afternoon staff dismissed them as *sundowning* and tried to distract her the best they knew how.

A conversation with her daughter revealed that for years Marge would pick up her young children from school every afternoon. This information certainly explained her outbursts around 3pm. We suspected that the stress of the move had activated her old body clock and sent her into this *altered reality*. In her mind, she was a young mother and her children were stranded in front of the school and this locked exit was preventing her from reaching them. No wonder she was panic-stricken and hysterical.

The Loving Lie: Once we understood Marge's history, it didn't take long for us to come up with the perfect *loving lie*. The following afternoon when Marge was once again pounding on the door, we told her that her friend would pick up all the children from school today. Marge reacted with immediate relief, reverted back to her "present" self, and readily accepted our invitation to join the others for tea.

We used our *loving lie* for the next couple of weeks until one afternoon when she seemed to have forgotten all about the school, the children, and the exit door. I took this as a sign that she finally felt safe in her new environment.

Sam still appeared entirely lucid and reasonable. You'd be likely to question why he needed to live in a secured memory care unit. He enjoyed long and intricate conversations but might suddenly blurt out a remark completely out of context. One day in the middle of such a chat he mentioned that the skeletons were still visiting in his room at night. Of course we asked him to talk about them. He wasn't scared, he said, but rather a bit annoyed because they glowed in the dark and he couldn't understand what they were saying and even how they could talk since they had no tongues. After discussing this with him for a bit, we decided it might be worth trying to hang a sign to hang in his room that said, "Skeletons not welcome here. Go away." Sam most likely had Lewy Bodies dementia. His hallucinations were not limited to night visions. One day, he apparently saw a beach in place of the nurse's station and at another time, the patio outside the dining room window had turned into a riding stable for him. In Sam's case, our *loving lie* was the sign posted for his intruders. Later he reported that his skeleton traffic had declined some, so maybe the sign had worked a little bit.

Robert had been a prisoner of war in the Korean conflict. He would suddenly panic that "they" were coming for him. Was he "reliving" actual events as an altered reality or was he having hallucinations? We never knew just which, but it didn't matter. Our only mission at those times was to help him feel safe again. At first we told him that we wouldn't let anything bad happen to him. That did not convince him, so we had to come up with something much more authoritarian. We unplugged the phone and pretended to make calls to CIA, FBI, and military police to confirm that Robert's whereabouts were top-secret and that he was safe.

A Wedding

Charlotte was a resident in the Alzheimer's wing of the facility where my friend Paul was activity director. Paul shared with me this *altered reality* experience: Charlotte had growing difficulties with communication and was increasingly withdrawing into her own world. Since she had first moved into the nursing home, she had gone from one obsession to another. At one point, she had fixated on germs - on her clothes, in her food, and on anybody who might touch her. At another time it was something outside one particular window visible only to her. Her fixations usually lasted only long enough for the staff to readjust their approaches to her "reality de jour."

However one obsession took hold of her and had grown more intense as time went on. It had seemed innocuous at first. Charlotte parked herself daily on a bench near the entrance. Whenever the doorbell rang, she would perk up. However when the visitor apparently was not the one she had expected she'd sink into noticeable disappointment. Over the weeks Charlotte spirit turned from sadness to grief and despair. She was increasingly seen weeping. Staff decided they had to do something. Because of her difficulties with communication, it took a concerted effort for them to discern that Charlotte's vigil at the door was for her beloved, who had assured her that he would be there any day now to marry her.

A conversation with her niece revealed that Charlotte had in fact never married and the niece had never heard of a pending or canceled wedding. None of this made any sense. They speculated that her sweetheart had gone off to war and never returned. Charlotte wasn't able to tell them anything beyond: "He's coming soon and then we'll be married." (Or at least the aides were pretty sure that's what she said.)

The staff tried all kinds of diversions: They cajoled, flattered, and tried to entice her with cookies and songs, but all to no avail. Charlotte remained indifferent to their efforts. The niece took her out to twice as many lunches as before, but as soon as they returned, Charlotte would resume her brooding vigil at the door. She changed. She had always been gentle and cooperative in spite of her obsessions and hallucinations. Now she was frequently agitated and obstinate.

Drastic measures were needed. Paul decided they would have to celebrate her "wedding." The staff readily committed to help make this happen. At a local thrift store, Paul found a wedding gown that promised a reasonably good fit. One of the nurses brought a bouquet of silk flowers from the front lobby. On the designated day, the staff rearranged the furniture and decorated the dining room, the kitchen baked a tiered "wedding" cake and family members, who happened to be visiting at the moment, were recruited to stay on as "wedding guests." Staff made sure that all the residents were dressed in their Sunday best.

Everything was in place except for the fiancé. What to do? So Paul decided to act as the stand-in for the groom. He pinned a showy white silk rose to the lapel of his coat. One of the other residents, a retired organist, played a pretty good simile of the wedding march. The bride beamed in all her finery as she was walked down the "aisle," on the arm of the cook. The janitor, a long scarf draped around his neck, performed the "ceremony." It was a glorious affair. The reception was the best party the nursing home had ever had.

Charlotte basked in the spotlight for the rest of the afternoon. By the next morning she seemed to have forgotten everything, but her demeanor had changed; she was calm and unperturbed. She didn't once go near the entrance. The subjects of fiancés and weddings never came up again. Nobody ever learned what event in Charlotte's life had bubbled to the surface because of the disease - or if this had been pure fantasy. But thanks to Paul's creativity, it apparently had been resolved for Charlotte. She was back to her contented and gentle self.

"I want to go home!"

Most residents are moved to a care facility when it's clear that it's no longer safe for them to live on their own. The individual wasn't eating right and spent the day in a nightgown. She no longer bathed or cleaned her house. It was obviously a necessary move and she ought to be happy that she was rescued, right? But she doesn't see it like that. As far as she's concerned, she was doing just fine in her own house and she gets very upset when we tell her that she can no longer take care of herself and she's *living here* now.

We can help people with transitioning into this new environment. First we want to be aware of our communication. *Living here* feels permanent and irrevocable. Try to replace it with *Staying here. Staying* is temporary and could mean a weekend or 10 years. It helps us to remember that leaving home and losing one's independence is as devastating as losing a loved one, and in this case your resident had no say in what happened to her.

If her home was sold to pay for her care, it's a topic best left alone. I've heard well-meaning family members, determined to *tell the truth,* say, "Your house was sold, so you can't go home." That truth can be so devastating that it may plunge a person into a deeper state of dementia and possibly bring on depression as well. It might help the family to sit in on care management meetings. It's important for everyone involved to understand the importance of using the same *loving lies.* If she asks directly about her house, you can tell her that everything is fine and someone you trust is taking care of it while she's *staying* here.

With "I want to go home," she may be thinking of her most recent home or she may be alluding to her childhood home. On the other hand her plea may have little to do with an actual location. She has lost her independence and freedom and she's feeling loss and anxiety at being in unfamiliar surroundings. Your reactions should be the same, either way. Your aim is to help her feel at home, i.e. emotionally safe.

She'll probably adjust in time, but in the meantime you'll have a better chance of gaining her trust if you tell her how glad you are that she's *visiting* with you and that you're glad to know her. If she continues to obsess about her own home, acknowledge her feelings, but don't linger on the topic; instead, try talking about things that she used to do in her home: You've heard that she's a great gardener (cook, ironer, silver polisher or whatever) and how you could use her help with some of those things while she's *staying* with you. Then, use it as a lead-in to a diversion: "Don't you think this conversation deserves a cup of tea?" or - "go for a walk," - "read this new magazine with me," - "help me with the cookies" – (or whatever fits the moment.) The point of this exchange is to help her feel included, safe, and validated.

Lolo had lived in our facility for seven years and yet she continued to believe that she's simply visiting for the weekend. One of our oft recurring conversations went like this:

> *Me:* Lolo, we sure had a great time today. I'll see you in a few days.
> *Lolo:* Probably not. I'm going home tomorrow.
> *Me:* Well, I hope to catch you before you go, okay?

Sometimes Lolo would add that she's had a very pleasant stay at this nice "hotel." - Nobody told her otherwise.

Sundowning or Body Clocks?

Many of us are sensitive to the waning light in late afternoon. When this affects people with Alzheimer's or related dementias, it's known as *sundown syndrome* or *sundowning.* In some cases *sundowning* causes agitation, a change in personality, or increased confusion. In cases of serious agitation diagnosed as *sundowning*, it is quite common to prescribe an anti-anxiety medication. Before we medicate people to change their behavior, I believe we need to explore other possibilities. In my experience more often than not, these behaviors have been reactions to people's internal body clocks possibly brought on by the waning light in the late afternoon.

Body Clocks. We all have more or less active body clocks. We wake up a few minutes before the alarm goes off - or we get antsy at dinnertime, whether we're hungry or not. Most of us spend most of our lives in regular routines. Just because a person has "retired" from a job that she held most of her life, doesn't necessarily mean her body is aware of her new life at leisure, so when it's close to her old *quitting time* she may have the urge to go home, or she may not feel complete until she has *closed the books, cleaned up her desk,* or *punched out.*

When the person exhibits changes in her behavior in the late afternoon, I recommend that you explore the possibility that she's reacting to old body clock impulses before assuming this to be *sundowning.* If you cannot identify an exact cause, try to use a diversion that relates to her former life: If she worked in an office, you can hand her a few files to organize or if she worked in retail give her a cash box with change to be counted. Whether or not she actually engages in the project, be sure to thank her for her help.

The following situation illustrates how easily circumstances can be mistaken for *sundowning*:

Ruth cheerfully participated in our activities. However, around 4 o'clock in the afternoon her personality changed. On better days she would simply be sullen and distant; on the worst days she would become restless, fidgety, and agitated, sometimes to the point of tears. This had been going on for weeks and everyone assumed that she was *sundowning* and beyond our help. We tried to distract her by getting her involved in activities. It might work for a few minutes, but before long she would be back pacing, usually around the serving counter in the kitchen area. Our common room, which also served as a dining room, was a converted apartment, so it had a kitchenette with a breakfast bar but all the meals were prepared in the main kitchen and brought down to us on individual plates. Ruth's agitation was primarily focused on the empty kitchen.

Because Ruth's behavior was so consistent, we decided to explore the body clock possibility. We learned that her husband was a stickler for rigid schedules and during the fifty-plus years of their marriage Ruth had served dinner daily at six o'clock sharp. Her agitation made sense. Ruth's body clock was on *"dinner fixing"* time. In her mind she needed to prepare the meal and there was nothing for her to work with. Ideally, we would have asked Ruth to help with food preparation, but unfortunately all the meals arrived fully prepared in the central kitchen. We did ask her to help set the table, but that only worked to accelerate her agitation.

The **Loving Lie:** We had to find another solution. We told Ruth that someone else was doing the cooking tonight, because she deserved a day off after all those years of making dinner every single night. She accepted our story with no hesitation. She welcomed the break, which was understandable; apparently her husband was quite controlling, including over her household.

Once we understood the reasons for Ruth's anxiety, we initiated preventative action. As soon as her demeanor started to shift, we would ask for her help in planning tomorrow's menu, while reminding her that she could take tonight off. Ruth's daughter got involved in our project as well. She brought gourmet magazines, a cookbook and a recipe file box. The two of them would find a corner table and talk up a storm. She helped Ruth write recipes on her index cards and cut out pictures of impossible delectables, which we kept in a *portfolio* (a manila folder with her name on it.)

After Ruth's passing, her daughter thanked us for giving her the best couple of years with her mom. Before the recipe project, it had been so hard for her to visit her beloved mother because she hadn't known what to talk about, which had been a constant reminder that her mother was fading away. Sharing something that they both genuinely enjoyed had brought back so much of the mom she used to know.

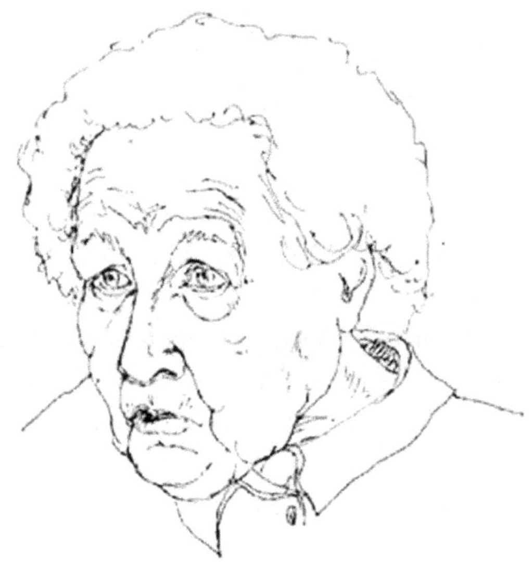

Memory, Lies, or Fantasy?

Every case of dementia is unique. For some people the decline is pretty steady, while many others experience a great deal of fluctuations and sudden declines followed by plateaus. One day a person appears pretty normal, the next she may not recognize even the most familiar.

This can be most disconcerting to family members. An otherwise loving wife may suddenly think that her husband of forty years is a dangerous intruder and try to chase him out of the house with a frying pan.

There's no predicting which memory will surface or vanish at any particular moment. She may suddenly have forgotten something that you reasonably considered totally familiar. Maybe she refuses to go to a store right down the street, telling you she doesn't know where it is. This is the same store where she has shopped for thirty years, so you may think she's lying to you or simply because she's lazy and doesn't want to get out of her chair.

She can likely tell by your tone of voice that she *should* know the answer, a realization that is probably terrifying to her. If you persist, she may get quite agitated or depressed and the rest of your day is easily ruined. However, if you start with the assumption that she's not trying to deceive you, but rather it's the disease surfacing, it will make life so much better for both of you. Take a few moments to

sit with her, share a refreshment and some good
innocuous chit-chat or "girl-talk." Give her time to
collect herself and relax. • Rule of thumb: stress
leads to confusion and memory loss.

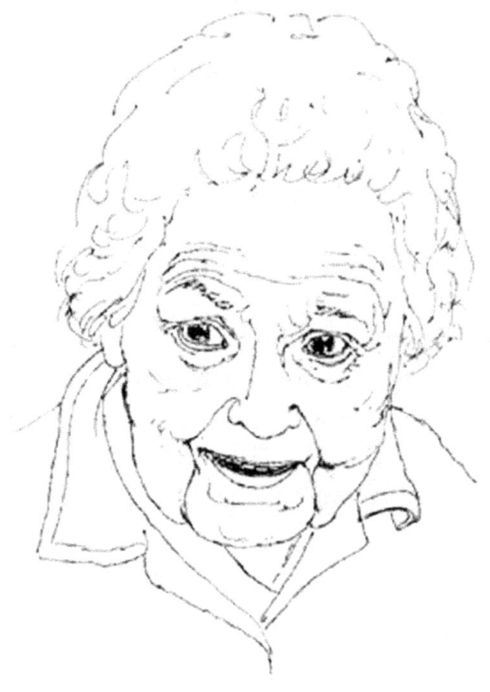

Most of us will sort stuff. Human beings apparently have a strong need to bring order to chaos and that's the secret to the success of fiddle boxes.

When a person is restless, pacing, or even agitated, you may be able to calm him by soliciting his help straightening out a fiddle box. It's important that you present it to him as a serious task that you need help with. When you sense that he feels that he's finished, you'll want to thank him – even if he's done nothing except simply look at it.

I use containers the size of a shoe box or smaller. A large box may be overwhelming and could defeat your purpose. Your friend may look at it and give up before she even starts. I also prefer a container that's light enough to carry around.

Fiddle box ideas:
- Post cards
- Clips from magazines
- Recipe file
- Playing cards
- Baking and cooking stuff: small wooden spoons, measuring cups, ladles, whisks
- Office stuff - small notepad, hole punch, erasers, pencils, paper clips
- Jewelry: long strands of beads in different colors, necklaces, pendants and clip-on

earrings (no rings or pins)
* Baby things: pacifiers, baby clothes, bottles, rattles, small stuffed toys
* Art supplies: dried tubes of paint with their caps super glued in place, crayons, brushes
* PVC pipe connections and safe small tools
* Packets of seeds, a garden catalog and plastic gardening tools
* Individual paint sample cards, (found on racks at a home improvement store)

Willie had reached the advanced stage of Alzheimer's disease. He was wheelchair bound and his ability to speak was pretty much gone. Most of his remaining vocabulary was limited to colorful curses, which he would practice loudly, especially whenever everyone else was having a lot of fun. We tried to get him involved in our activities to no avail.

When we learned that he used to own a thriving business as a supplier of custom and high-end windows and doors, we created a box for him with 20 –30 pictures of windows and doors cut out of decorator magazines. Soon he would pull out the pictures one by one and lay them out on the table, methodically sorting them by size, style etc.

Elaine was a nurse - retired as far as the system was concerned. However she was nowhere ready to hang it up. Physically she was in great shape, but unfortunately her dementia had affected her mental functions and her mind was in a constant turmoil.

She had a very hard time when she was moved into our Alzheimer's facility. We had very little to satisfy her need for a purpose. Based on what we learned about her past, we filled her box with bandages, rubber gloves, cotton balls, tongue depressors, etc - you get the point. We also gave her black and red ballpoint pens, a clipboard with a chart and a name tag with her name and: *Assistant Nurse*. Our nurse at the time played right along and when Elaine was restless or anxious, she would solemnly ask for Elaine's help writing down the vitals as they were doing rounds.

Alvina had her first morning at our facility. Apparently there had been no attempt to help her with a gentle transition. She was understandable very angry. Her loss of language (aphasia) only aggravated her agitation. Alvina was a large woman, so when she started swinging at the staff and other residents, we needed a distraction instantly. I grabbed the closest item at hand, which happened to be a box of several hundred crayons, old and new, all colors and at different stages of wear. Admittedly, I was as concerned as everyone else, so I took a deep breath to disguise my apprehension as I handed her the box and as calmly as possible said, "Hi Alvina, it's so good to meet you. – I hear that you're great at organizing stuff. I sure could use your help with this box. Would you mind helping me sort it out?" Alvina stopped abruptly, looked at me and then focused on the box and nodded with a half smile. I placed the box on a table in the dining room and pulled the chair out for her. She immediately started laying out the crayons. Two hours later it was lunchtime, but she was still at it and we didn't dare to interrupt her for fear that her agitation would return, so we rearranged the seating in the room. She continued happily until she had hundreds of crayons very neatly laid out by color, tone and length in a beautiful pattern.

Kathleen was easily overwhelmed by our group projects. We knew she had an affinity for sparkles and jewels and I happened to have a collection of inexpensive costume jewelry, including a number of necklaces and half a dozen long strands of "pearls" (sold by the foot at the hobby store.) I created a special fiddle box for her. She dove right into the tangled mess and started sorting them out. It was the most engaged she had been in a long time. From then whenever she started to show agitation, we would hand her the box and ask her to help us sort it out. She would find a quiet corner and start making designs out of swirled strands. This kept her happily occupied daily for well over a year.

Ethel's daughter called me excitedly: "I can't believe it – Mother sang all the way to the doctor's office and back!" The daughter continued, "I don't know when and where she learned all of those songs. There was no music in the house when I grew up, no radio, no record player, no dancing and no singing."

I had never known that side of Ethel. By the time I met her she was already in the mid-stage of Alzheimer's. Her speech was halting and her thoughts definitely fractured, but she loved to sing. Now, two or three years later, she could no longer hold up a conversation, but she still sang. She sang in the shower; she sang on our walks; she hummed to herself while working on projects in our arts and crafts sessions. Ethel sang to me, to the cat, to the flowers in the garden, and to other residents. She was one of the kindest and most generous of our residents, always ready to cheer others up.

As soon as she would start to sing, the aphasia was gone. The lyrics flowed effortlessly and she hardly ever missed a word. This is the same woman who couldn't remember from five minutes ago and often didn't recognize her own children. Her repertoire seemed endless. Whereas I needed my songbooks, she had hundreds of songs memorized. I dreaded to think of what must have been going on in her life for her to have deprived her children of music in their home. Whatever it was, had completely vanished now that she was in the later stages of Alzheimer's, - one of the blessings of this dreaded disease.

Melinda and I developed a ritual that we practiced before every sing-along. I would fetch her with: "Melinda, please come join our sing-along. We really need your voice." - Without fail, Melinda would say: "You don't want me, I sound like a frog." To which I would respond with: "Hey, every singing group needs at least one frog." She would laugh and sing with gusto, albeit off key (or as we call it: *creative harmony*.) This scenario was repeated at every session for the six-plus years that she participated in our weekly sing-alongs.

Music and Memory Project. One of the most exciting recent happenings in eldercare is the *Music and Memory Project*. Thousands of elders in nursing homes are given iPods with their own favorite music. It's amazing to watch as they go from being locked into their silent worlds to being completely connected and back to life as soon as they put on the headphones.

Q. My mother thinks I'm her sister. It breaks my heart that she no longer knows who I am.

A. When your mom mistakes you for her sister or mother, it's obvious that she recognizes you as a person whom she trusts and loves. Your willingness to be accepted as these different people will give you the valuable opportunity to learn more about Mom, not only who she is as your mother, but who she is as a human being.

Q. Do all Alzheimer patients get the negative attitude?

A. The "negative" attitude of People with Alzheimer's or similar memory-impairment is often caused by the mood, tone and attitude of their caregivers. Because of their disorders, their impressions and perceptions are easily distorted and influenced by external factors. When we set a positive tone, we'll get a positive reaction. The "negative" attitude may be caused by the frustration at not being able to make oneself understood.

Q. I'm caring for my mother. My brother is charge of her finances; I'm constantly having to explain things to him. but he lives in another state. Although he phones her every week, he hasn't seen Mom in person in over a year, so he doesn't understand the situation,

A. Sadly, this is a common situation. As a rule of thumb it's advisable that whoever lives nearest to the parent holds the POA for healthcare. Crucial decisions often must be made at the spur of the moment.

Distant Relatives.
Susannah is a family caregiver caring for her mother at home. Her brother lives halfway across the country. For the last year, his only contact with their mother has been phone conversations where he does all the talking and mom responds in simple platitudes; consequently he has very distorted impressions of the situation and has relentlessly questioned Susannah's assessment of mom's condition. As happens in many families, as the son, he was designated the agent in charge of the mother's finances. He's constantly questioned every expense submitted for reimbursement. Fortunately she managed to convince him to fly out to stay with mom while she took a short vacation. She returned to find her brother exhausted and with a new appreciation for her daily life.

Q. *My father lives in an Alzheimer's home. My mom visits him every week. The other day, she walked in on him hugging and kissing another resident. She was horribly shaken and crying when she called me.*

A. **Love Nest.**
A care facility contacted me about a similar issue. One of their male residents was spending a lot of time cuddling with a female resident, much to the distress of his wife. They weren't sure if they should move him into a different wing to keep them apart. After talking for a bit we agreed that the issue was not with the resident but rather the wife needing to understand that this behavior had nothing to do with her relationship with him We talked about *Residents' Rights*, self-determination and basic emotional needs. A successful care facility strives to achieve a feeling of family among its residents and staff, so affection becomes a natural component. It's not uncommon for residents in facilities to develop deep affection for each other. Spouses may visit daily for an hour, two, or even four out of twenty-four.

One of my colleagues tells me that her facility is often a veritable Peyton Place with several couples and threesomes. These trysts definitely enliven the place and bring joy to those involved. She tells me the difficulties arise when a visiting spouse gets upset at this. That's understandable. We work hard to help the spouse understand that dementia in the advanced stages frequently causes the person to forget the nature of relationships within the family. Daughters are confused with wives and wives are mistaken for mothers or sisters. Importantly, there's almost always a recognition of a loving bond with a family member.

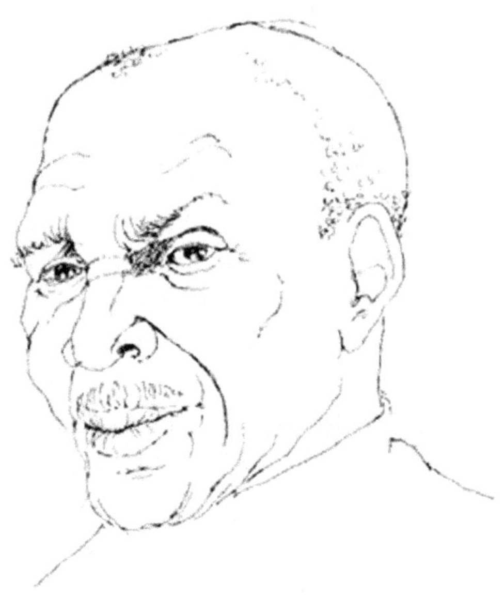

Dementia Basics Quiz

*Please remember that these behaviors are caused by a
disease whether it's Alzheimer's or another dementia
What would you do in these situations?*

1. *Ed will not sit down for a meal.*
a. Give him finger food to eat while he's pacing.
b. Tell him to sit down, because he's upsetting others.
c. Tie him to his seat so he can't get up.

2. *Jane insists that she must go home.*
a. Remind her she lives here now.
b.Tell her to stop, because she's disturbing other people.
c. Ask her to help you with something.

3. *Paul refuses to shower.*
a. Have two of you walk him to the shower.
b. Firmly tell him he has to take his bath now.
c. Tell him you promised to help him and right now is a good time.

4. *Hal is walking down the hallway without a stitch of clothes on. What would you say to him?*
a. "What are you thinking, being out here naked?"
b. "It's really too cold not to wear clothes. I'll be glad to help you get dressed."
c. "Go back to your room right now and get dressed!"

5. *Victor has been peeing in his trashcan.*
    a. Tell him that it's nasty to pee in the trashcan.
    b. Make a big sign: BATHROOM with an arrow
    c. Remove his trashcan.

6. *Carol believes there's a bear in her closet.*
    a. Tell her it's her imagination-there is no bear.
    b. Pretend to lead the bear out of the room.
    c. Ask that she be moved to another room.

7. *Linda's staring at her food without eating a bite.*
    a. She wants special attention and someone to feed her.
    b. She may have a low-grade infection, i.e. a UTI or her gums or teeth may be hurting.
    c. She's confused by too much food on her plate requiring different utensils.

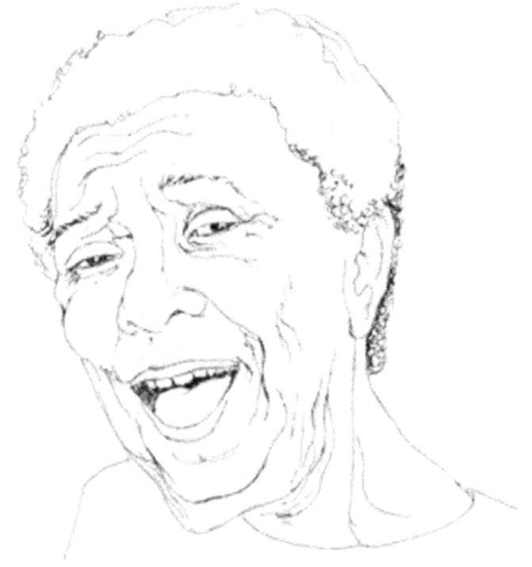

Solutions

1. – A. *Ed's pacing is caused by the disease and even if he wanted to, he probably cannot stop pacing. Every time he passes by you, give him a bitesized piece of "fingerfood." Make sure to give him lots of water and extra calories.*

2. – C. *Words matter:* **Living** *is longterm or permanent, whereas* **staying** *is temporary, it can be for the afternoon or a month or a year. Tell Jane how glad you are that she's* **staying** *with you and find something she can help you with.*

3. – C. *Paul will get very angry if two of you try to force him against his will. When you tell him that you promised him, giving him the sense of control over his life.*

4. – B. *Most importantly, act normal. Try to find out why Hal has taken off his clothes. Is something binding, itchy or irritating to his skin or is he too hot? Or did he have an "accident" and didn't know how to get dressed again? – If this happens frequently, one solution is to have him wear onesies that zip up the back, so he can't undress by himself.*

5. – B. *Most likely Victor can't find the bathroom and he doesn't want to soil the floor, so he's found a container to use as a potty. Put up signs with arrows pointing toward the bathroom. OR he has declining eyesight and with everything white in the bathroom he simply cannot distinguish the toilet from the floor. Solution: a toilet seat in contrasting color.*

6. – B. *Carol may have* **Lewy Body Disease** *and she may be prone to hallucinations. The bear is REAL to her. Moving her to another room is not likely to change anything. The best solution is to enter into her perception and "lead the bear out of the room" and then follow-up with a diversion that she enjoys.*

7. – B and C *Linda is not doing this intentionally. If this is happening suddenly, chances are that she's not feeling well. Or she may be confused about how to use her utensils. There may be too many choices on her plate. First try to offer her a smaller portion that requires only one utensil. You can also try using a smaller plate – preferably red (stimulates the appetite.) You may also try to "model" for her by eating with her. Watching you eat may spur her or remind her of what to do.*

<u>Understanding Dementia and Alzheimer's</u>

The Nun Study (early study on Alzheimer's)
<u>http://www.healthstudies.umn.edu/nunstudy/</u>
The first solid evidence of the importance of
keeping our brains stimulated.

**Decoding Darkness, The Search for the Genetic
Causes of Alzheimer's Disease**
by Rudolph E. Tanzi and Ann B. Parson
<u>http://www.amazon.com/Decoding-
Darkness-Genetic-Alzheimers-Disease/dp/
0738205265</u>
This fascinating reveal of the scientific
research industry reads like a detective story..

Experience Alzheimer's
<u>https://www.youtube.com/watch?v=LL_Gq7Shc-Y</u>
Virtual dementia tour

Living with Dementia, incl. Alzheimer's
Richard Taylor, Ph.D.
<u>http://www.richardtaylorphd.com/blog/</u>
<u>http://
www.bestdementiavideosandbooks.com/
products_detail.php?ProductID=3</u>
Videos of Richard Taylor, Ph.D
https://www.youtube.com/watch?v=lHQfc3KJ9qE

<u>The Pioneers, and Innovators</u>

The Pioneer Network
<u>http://Pioneernetwork.net</u>

The Dementia Action Alliance
<u>http://daanow.org/</u>

It's Their Life
<u>http://www.cbc.ca/player/Radio/</u>
<u>The+Sunday+Edition/ID/2304600853/</u>

Dementia Village NL:
<u>https://www.youtube.com/watch?</u>
<u>v=LwiOBlyWpko</u>
<u>http://www.cnn.com/2013/07/11/world/</u>
<u>europe/wus-holland-dementia-village/</u>
<u>http://www.aplaceformom.com/blog/</u>
<u>pioneering-dementia-care-facility/</u>

San Luis Obispo Helping Hands handmade soap project:
<u>https://www.youtube.com/watch?</u>
<u>v=nE1A5SLqHro</u>
<u>https://www.youtube.com/watch?</u>
<u>v=G9r5sVbZOx4</u>

Through the Looking Glass II
<u>http://www.illinoispioneercoalition.org/</u>
<u>news/detail.php?id=2</u>

Dr G. Allen Power
<u>http://www.alpower.net/</u>
<u>gallenpower_bio.htm</u>

Dr. Bill Thomas:

http://changingaging.org
http://thegreenhouseproject.org/

Teepa Snow

Books, programs, DVDs:
http://teepasnow.com/

Gary Glazner

The Alzheimer's Poetry Project
http://www.alzpoetry.com/

Anne Bastings

TimeSlips writing and storytelling project
https://www.timeslips.org/

Virtual Memory Cafés

Online meeting place
https://www.dementiamentors.org/virtual
memory-cafes.html

<u>**Finding a nursing home**</u>

> https://www.medicare.gov/
> nursinghomecompare/search.html

Ombudsman - We recommend that you acquaint yourself with the Ombudsman volunteer at the facility.

From their official website: *Long-term care ombudsmen are advocates for residents of nursing homes, board and care homes and assisted living facilities. Ombudsmen provide information about how to find a facility and what to do to get quality care. They are trained to resolve problems. If you want, the ombudsman can assist you with complaints. However, unless you give the ombudsman permission to share your concerns, these matters are kept confidential. Under the federal Older Americans Act, every state is required to have an Ombudsman Program that addresses complaints and advocates for improvements in the long-term care system.*

Facilities are required to display posters featuring "Residents' Rights" with information on how to contact the Ombudsman.

www.ingramcontent.com/pod-product-compliance
Lightning Source LLC
Chambersburg PA
CBHW061035050726
47592CB00004B/1449